Ultimate WEIGHT LOSS Blueprint After 30

Ultimate

WEIGHT LOSS

Blueprint After 30

Luis Felipe Ninja Pinto

Bachelor of Science

4 x World Champion in Brazilian Jiu Jitsu

ISBN: 978-1-964913-70-4 (Paperback)

Printed in the United States of America

Contents

Foreword

Hello, My name is Luis Felipe Ninja Pinto. I come from Sao Paulo, Brazil, and I currently reside in Kansas City. As the proud founder of a Martial Arts School teaching various different styles of combat sports such as Brazilian Jiu-Jitsu, Capoeira and Muay Thai, I believe that I can make a difference in the lives of people through the teaching of these arts as well as providing knowledge that can help them lead healthier lives. We live in a dangerous world where it's imperative to understand how to defend yourself, and aside from the utilitarian usage of these arts I believe that the discipline that they inculcate within a person can help people lead fulfilling lives. I am a family man and am married to my wife Renata and have three kids Kaue, Yuri and Yara. Beyond my children and my wife, my family includes my cherished mother, Lola and my brother, Henrique. We are a tight-knit unit as a family, and through mutual support and shared experiences, we navigate through the chaos of life. This book is a glimpse of my family and provides an idea of the various dynamics and the interplay that happens when you combine a Brazilian living in the ever-changing world of Kansas City. My journey is one filled with martial arts, strong family ties and raising a loving family.

Hitting 30 can be overwhelming. Your body just isn't the same as it used to be when you were younger, and you just aren't the same. Once I hit 30, I discovered the key to staying in shape. I'm not trying to sell you on some magic pill or fancy secret. It's just a simple method I developed after learning from highly qualified doctors and scientists. The whole journey began years ago, back in 2010, when I was having a difficult time with my family. My father had a Pancreatic cancer diagnosis, and it hit the entire family really hard. My dad was my hero, the soccer and life coach and also the glue that was binding the family together. I tried to save him, and in my desperate attempt, I dove headfirst into learning the intricacies of nutrition and diet to see what could possibly make a difference.

The cancer was relentless; my father underwent a 13-hour surgery, and even that wasn't enough. I researched whatever I could, ranging from clinical trials to medical books. I even bought some questionable medication from Mexico. Unfortunately, my father lost his battle against cancer and passed away in November 2010. However, I was not ready to give up.

In my research, I discovered that sugar was fuel for cancer cells, and the real path forward was to completely remove carbs from our diets and to become fat-adapted. The ketogenic diet, so to speak. I discovered that processed carbs and sugar were the main cause of metabolic disorders such as type 2 diabetes, obesity and, in general, bad eating habits.

I experimented with various diets. I tried the vegetarian diet, carnivore, and ketogenic, and I even tried the fast food American diet, if you can believe it. This showed me what works and, more importantly, what does not work. Once I discovered what the proper human diet needs to be, I cracked the code to longevity and health. I was able to easily make weight for Martial arts tournaments, and my sense of well-being skyrocketed.

I've tested these methods on friends, family, students and many others. The result? People lose a tremendous amount of weight, in some cases almost up to 80 pounds, simply by following my advice. Even my dog, Bella, was able to live an impressive 13 years following my diet, which is considered a very long life for a mastiff.

This is going to be a transformative journey but to understand it, let's dive deep into the essence of real food. Imagine you find yourself in the heart of the Amazon rainforest, a place free from modern supermarkets and rampant consumerism. Here, you won't find cereals, cookies or pasta. This tells you something very important: our bodies function their best on the nutrition provided by nature, not the artificially processed nutrition that permeates the contemporary world.

Processed food is a far-recent phenomenon in terms of human evolution. Our bodies and the way they function have not entirely become attuned to these edible products. And many of these products are not even real food. This is why they simply destroy our health. Imagine giving a lion a diet of pastries and sodas. The lion would become sick and die. We, as humans, aren't that far off.

This book will unravel the secrets of what a genuine, natural diet looks like. The journey begins with steering away from the processed junk food that we encounter in our daily lives and reclaiming our health and vitality. Along the way we'll uncover the secret to sustaining a healthy life, into and beyond our 30's.

I've experienced incredible transformations in the lives of many different people. This entire journey is about embracing change and becoming in tune with our biological needs. This book will teach you how to eat well, live a healthy life and thrive regardless of age. Let's learn the truth about the ideal human diet!

Introduction

This book contains the specifics of how individuals over 30 can implement life changing principles effectively to both achieve their weight loss goals and improve their health and well-being.

I share this wisdom of healthy weight loss with you because I feel that I can help other people improve their lives, much like I improved mine. I grew up eating practically anything, and everything that tasted good, and as a Brazilian, the vibrant cuisine we have was my dietary weakness. My mother, with her amazing culinary skills, has always had a knack for crafting the most exquisite desserts I have ever tasted. I hold no experience in coaching, so much of the information I have now comes from my own experience with the ketogenic diet and the lessons I have learned along the way.

However, I am not a medical professional, whatever advice I do give is not medical advice. If you are an individual with a pre-existing condition, I would advise you to consult with your healthcare provider before attempting to make a significant dietary or lifestyle change. This book is simply based on my personal journey and what has worked for me and many other people.

This whole journey is going to be about empowerment. A journey of growth, development and taking back control of your life and health. I'm here to lead you to a better future. And you can always reach out to me for assistance or consultation at ninjapinto@gmail.com.

Chapter 1

Embracing Change: Navigating Weight Loss After 30

Life is all about change, and humans have evolved to adapt to change. Our bodies were designed by nature to adapt to difficult and ever-changing conditions, and as a result, we have dominated the world and become the leading species. When you, as an individual, embark on a journey of self-improvement and growth, you witness a change within you, making a change as transformative as this affects you on a very deep level. You gain a greater degree of confidence, discovering a new version of yourself.

The biggest change that comes from witnessing fat loss results are confidence and a positive self-perception. When you start seeing changes in the mirror and noticing that clothes fit you better, you become much more confident and happier as an individual. It helps that it also makes the diet easier to follow when you know that it's working.

Every pound you lose, every inch that falls off your waist, is a milestone, and it helps encourage you to keep moving forward. With every day, you see changes that push you toward your ideal body shape, and that is what gives you the confidence and the positive reinforcement to keep moving forward.

To understand why this diet works, it's imperative to understand how the body functions in terms of metabolism and physiology. There exists an interplay between diet, hormone levels, moods and energy. It's entirely possible to manipulate these variables to our advantage.

Discipline is paramount to begin your journey of transformation. Without discipline, you will find yourself falling off the wagon more often than not. There will be days when you lack the motivation to keep moving forward to stick with your diet. You'll have ideas such as "Maybe if I can cheat today, I can make up for it tomorrow", but this is precisely what holds progress back. This is why my book holds an entire chapter on discipline and cultivating it.

This path of health and wellness is one that's been shaped by my family, my passions and my father's cancer diagnosis. This path is deeply personal to me, and I want everyone to be able to live life to their fullest with the information I will provide.

Growing up, I was a very athletic young man. I played a lot of soccer and even gained a scholarship due to it. However, my real passion was martial arts, Capoeira and Brazilian Jiu-jitsu mainly. I started learning capoeira in 1992 and I was very into all the flips and acrobatic moves of the art. Brazilian Jiu-Jitsu came into my life in 1998. Combat sports are very grueling, and to compete in a tournament, you have to "make weight", cutting a lot of weight to fit into a weight category. I'd work tirelessly in the gym, ensuring that I burnt more calories than I ate. Every training session was more brutal than the last and I suffered for my sport. I loved the sport and the arts, and as a result, I have taught many people martial arts and even held seminars on the sports, meeting many new people along the way.

My life took a turn when my father was diagnosed with pancreatic cancer, and my focus was then shifted towards learning various applications of how diet could improve his life. I tried to find a miracle, but I couldn't, and it was unfortunately too late for my father. I didn't stop learning. However, I tried to understand how to prevent cancer from occurring and in my research, I one day had a conversation with a friend and fellow capoeira teacher, Dr Chad Adams, who suggested something that would seem contradictory to hear, "What if you could lose fat by eating mostly fat?"

An idea that sounds preposterous at first glance, but when I delved deeper into the research, the books and the articles, I discovered something profound. The more I learned about this unconventional method, the more intrigued I became, and when I experimented with a ketogenic diet, I was astonished by the results. I was able to easily achieve my fitness goals, and I also found myself coaching and guiding family members, friends, students and even strangers who needed my help.

14 years later, I believe I have cracked the code to health, performance and vitality. I learned to help myself as well as others around me. I even helped a few diabetics to be able to live life without needing insulin shots. My own mother, who had thyroid issues, lost 40 pounds.

This book will contain many stories and transformations of people who, much like me, embarked on this amazing journey. These people are more than just friends. They're family. We are all bound by this uplifting change that we have experienced in our lives. Health and wellness have completely shifted the course of our lives.

It is important to remember that it all begins when you make that decision, to embrace change and to become better, every single step forward, every milestone, brings greater confidence.

The journey will be difficult, but it will be rewarding. Everyone doubted me or thought I was crazy, but I made it work for me, and I know you will, too, when you embark on this powerful and transformative path.

I'll give a personal anecdote that shows the effectiveness of this method. My wife doubted my eating habits throughout. Her turning point came when she gave birth to our twins and became self-conscious about her post-pregnancy stomach. She considered liposuction to remove the extra skin, but that's where I came in and told her that if she just gave me eight weeks, if she didn't see a difference, I would personally pay for her liposuction. She agreed to try my methods, and I am proud to say that she has now reclaimed the body of her youth. The transformation went far beyond just the physical it was a transformation of the mind and the soul as well.

So, with all that said, this will be a powerful and transformational journey for you. You will grow as a person and see a massive change in your own life. More than just the weight loss and the physical changes.

Chapter 2

Nutrition Reset: Crafting a Balanced Eating Plan

Some things you need to consider before delving into the ketogenic diet. Firstly, the way our ancestors navigated the world is a far cry from how we do things. The diets that they consumed were out of necessity and also shaped by the environment they found themselves in. The foods they ate were not eaten out of convenience but rather based on one thing and one thing only: survival. These eating instincts and principles overlap with the ketogenic diet.

Our ancestors would often go on days without food, fasting and eating when they could rather than having a fixed schedule of meals. We are not that different from our ancestors. You have to keep in mind, for example, why do we NEED to eat breakfast in the morning? We don't need to. We just do it because, apparently, "breakfast is the most important meal of the day," or so we're told. It's not. There is no specific meal that's so important. We're supposed to eat when we're truly hungry, not when we're 'craving' something. Going back to the point about our ancestors, they ate when they needed to. The rest of the time, they would go through periods of no food and just water. This led to metabolic processes and adaptations that allow for the person to enter a state known as ketosis. Ketosis is the state wherein stored fat becomes the primary energy source, rather than glucose/glycogen, which is the energy stored in muscles.

Entering the world of fasting was an exciting journey. I felt as if I was traversing uncharted territory. The idea of eating only once in a 24-hour period seemed, quite frankly, insane to someone like me. As a competitive athlete, we were taught to eat multiple times a day, consume supplements and often have a large pre-competition meal that would be usually filled to the brim with carbs such as pasta. How wrong I was.

A lot of my ideas on diet were based on common misconceptions. I also discovered that many of the problems I had during training, such as the weakness and dizziness I felt, were due to a lack of hydration rather than calories. This was a big revelation for me.

Once I started managing my electrolyte intake during the fasting periods I was going on, I began to understand the importance of hydration as well as electrolyte intake. Once these problems were rectified, my dizziness and weakness died off. Hydration is key for training, this ensures that the body holds on to adequate amounts of glycogen in the muscles. Water is more important than calories for athletic endeavors.

I basically discovered that a body fat percentage starting from 12% was sufficient enough to fuel me through even the most grueling and difficult training sessions. This is because 12% and above body fat tend to have enough fat in the body to convert to energy for working out. Once I discovered this, I understood the human body's powerful capabilities.

Fasting was a very common occurrence for our ancestors. It was honestly just a way of life for them. This meant that they had to utilize unique and innovative ways to keep hydration up and avoid dizziness and weakness. Nature presented them with solutions. Firstly, there were rocks that were rich in minerals, and so our forebears would lick these stones to obtain crucial electrolytes, mainly sodium, potassium and also magnesium. This was an ingenious method to maintain hydration in the absence of regular meals.

Our ancestors were very reliant on fat as a source of fuel in their diet. Fat is one of the only macronutrients that is highly dense in energy, holding a total of 9 calories per gram of fat compared to 4 for Carbohydrates and 4 for protein. This allowed them to alleviate hunger pangs throughout the day. Our ancestors were able to understand that and this allowed them to go through days without eating unhindered by feelings of intense hunger. This is a sensation that modern science has also understood and validated.

Our ancestors' diets contain within them immense wisdom. The ketogenic diet combined with fasting is something that is very natural to us as humans. Much of the modern interpretation of the ketogenic diet is inspired by the hunter-gatherer lifestyle of our ancestors and their dietary principles that allowed them to survive and thrive in a world hostile to them.

We must never forget our evolutionary history. Over time, modern solutions to age-old problems have made us forget where we started. If we have a problem and can't find the answers to it, there's a large chance that someone somewhere has been in our shoes, experienced it and dealt with it in the past. That's the beauty of history. You get to learn from the lessons of other people who came before us.

Chapter 3

Metabolism Unveiled: Understanding Your Body's Engine

Weight loss, done in a sustainable way after 30, is quite a journey. Let's look at how metabolism affects our bodies when it comes to the consumption of carbohydrates, proteins and fats. All of these essential macronutrients affect our bodies differently, and most of all, the way the ketogenic diet influences our glycemic index will provide us with a fresh perspective on dealing with long-term sustainable weight loss.

Carbohydrates originate from grains, fruits, and vegetables. They serve as the primary fuel source for our body. They are broken down into glucose, which is a rapid energy source. Sounds good, right? The problem is the rapid spike in blood sugar tha accompanies high-carb meals. This rapid spike leads to fluctuations in mood, energy levels and satiety or lack thereof.

Proteins build muscle; they are the building blocks of life and are located in meats, dairy, and legumes, and they are necessary for the repair and growth of muscles. Proteins also increase and promote a feeling of satiety and fullness. Unlike carbs, proteins slowly release glucose into the bloodstream, usually through a process known as gluconeogenesis. This is a much less efficient method of glucose uptake and is much slower than carbohydrates. However, the beauty of this process is that it's much more stable as compared to the ups and downs of carbohydrates.

The ketogenic diet utilizes a high amount of fats, moderate amounts of protein and trace or minimal amounts of carbs. The idea is to drastically reduce carb intake. This leads to the body utilizing its own fat stores instead of burning glucose for energy. This metabolic state is known as ketosis, and it encourages the body to use stored fat for energy, which promotes fat loss.

The glycemic index refers to the rate at which foods increase blood sugar levels. They are a key player in affecting our body's metabolism. The ketogenic diet reduces the glycemic load on our bodies. This leads to steady blood sugar levels and reduces insulin spikes as well as reducing the risk of crashing energy levels and intense cravings for more food. Ever notice how you crave more food after having Chinese takeout? It's simply due to the fact that Chinese food is notoriously high in carbs, this means the food is just not very satisfying and fulfilling.

The ketogenic diet offers a different approach to weight loss and health. It increases satiety, gradual weight loss and sheds off fat like it was never supposed to be there. The idea behind the ketogenic diet is simple: you are what you eat, and not all calories are created equal. Calories from carbs simply don't fill the body the same way that calories from fats do. This is why, on the ketogenic diet we consume the most satiating foods that are available: healthy fats and proteins.

Chapter 4

The Power of Portion Control: Eating Smarter, Not Less

This journey is all about learning about the ketogenic diet balance of macronutrients as well as the unique ability of intermittent fasting to provide stable and consistent energy throughout the day.

It is imperative to maintain a delicate balance of macronutrients to properly follow the ketogenic diet. The lion's share of macros in the keto diet are fats, which are supposed to be about 70-75% of the daily caloric intake, and protein follow second with 20-25%, and carbohydrates make up a tiny fraction at 5-10%.

Intermittent fasting makes it far easier to exhaust stored glucose within the muscles, and this allows us to enter a metabolic state of burning fat instead of glucose (the primary source of energy in most people) for energy. This is the primary mechanism of Ketosis.

It's not just about what one is eating. It's also about when one eats. Less frequent meals with enough calories allow one to utilize keto to its fullest. This is because it maintains your energy levels and allows you to reap all the metabolic benefits of the diet.

A very common diet in the mainstream is eating frequent smaller meals, each portion being smaller than the last. This approach is a way people think can trick the body into burning more calories; however, it only ends up doing the opposite as eating more frequent meals can cause the metabolism to slow down as well as lead to an increase in lethargy and sluggishness inadvertently causing more weight gain.

To create a transformation, it is necessary to nurture one's metabolism rather than manipulate it. The path to achieving this lofty goal is through the ketogenic diet and intermittent fasting. This is a lifestyle that matches up with the human biological rhythm.

These percentages mentioned previously are meant to be the key to attaining the perfect macronutrient balance that unlocks ketosis and, thus, the potential of your body.

The following chapters will guide you toward practical strategies that will offer insights into creating meals that boost your metabolism. Every bite and every fast will fuel your body and help it transform.

Let us look at the foods that aid your journey, as well as the fasting strategies that will help you attain ketosis.

Fats include avocados, olive oil, and nuts. These will be the basis upon which you power your body. The ketogenic diet also allows for certain carbohydrates, namely vegetables such as spinach, cauliflower, and zucchini. Proteins consist of meats and eggs that allow you to build muscle and repair them, too.

Intermittent fasting is a practice that allows one to enter ketosis much faster. The strategy employed should be a 16:8 one; this means that one would fast for 16 hours and eat within an 8-hour window. This is closer to biological metabolic rhythms and also helps promote ketosis.

Just like fasting for 16 hours gets one closer to ketosis easier, another strategy that takes one even deeper into ketosis is the 24-hour fast. This is an approach under which one abstains from eating for a whole day. This involves prolonged fasting that completely exhausts the glucose stores and leads your body to tap into stored fat for fuel.

It is essential that while fasting and trying to attain ketosis, the body must be nourished with the right foods, such as grilled chicken, some roasted vegetables, and a bit of olive oil. This allows you to fuel your body's needs while honoring keto principles.

The foods one chooses and the timing of the meals will help shape one's metabolism, whether it's fasting for 16 hours and eating for 8 or the 24-hour fast. Either method encourages fat burning and improves mental clarity and energy levels.

The foods you eat and the fasting strategies that are adopted intentionally bring you closer to a healthier version of yourself. The next few chapters will delve into the practical methods of meal prep to help prepare for a menu that will align with your goals.

It is now time to become a better version of yourself. Let's now look into how the hormone insulin affects our body and how it might be the most important hormone for fat loss.

Chapter 5

Hydration and Hormones: Keys to Sustainable Weight Loss

Insulin plays a massive role in weight gain, as well as how fasting affects one's insulin levels and recovery. Hydration during fasting was a personal victory I had while fasting and competing in Brazilian jiu-jitsu.

Insulin is essentially the hormone that regulates how glucose enters the cells for energy or storage. Consuming carbs, particularly sugary ones, spikes blood sugar, which triggers an insulin release. High insulin levels can lead to fat storage, which contributes to weight gain. Understanding how insulin affects our bodies is essential for managing weight.

Fasting is an important strategy that plays a powerful role in managing insulin and its effects. Fasting during any sort of split, be it 16:8 or 24 hours, is imperative, and it is imperative to pay attention to hydration. Fasting can cause dehydration, as food is how we provide our bodies with water. Proper hydration ensures optimal body function and supports the metabolic shift induced by fasting.

However, fasting is more than the simple intake of water; electrolytes from sodium, potassium, and magnesium play a key role in maintaining the ideal fluid balance and proper muscle function. During a fast, the body needs to replenish electrolytes to avoid dizziness, fatigue, and muscle cramps.

On a personal note, during the 2018 IBJJF No-Gi Worlds, I had undertaken a 5-day fast, simply relying on electrolytes for sustenance and as a result, I won first place. That is the power of proper hydration in enhancing performance as well as resilience.

Dizziness or weakness during a fast stems from a lack of hydration rather than food. As fasting depletes electrolytes, our bodies struggle to maintain balance. Embracing electrolyte-rich sources and staying well hydrated can counter these feelings of weakness and allow one to pass through periods with energy.

Intermittent fasting can be quite effective and healthy when one has more than 15% body fat. This is the point where the body has ample reserves to utilize during fasting periods to promote stability as well as well-being.

Upon the conclusion of this chapter, you must understand that the influence of insulin, as well as the power of fasting, is one that you can utilize to your advantage. With this knowledge, you will be able to make choices that will guide you to a better future. Whatever solution you utilize to manage your insulin, further chapters will delve even deeper into these dynamics to help you achieve your goals.

This entire journey is more than just losing fat. It's about understanding the balance that exists within the body and nourishing it with the ideal macro and micronutrients. This will help shape your well-being and allow for greater vitality.

Chapter 6

Moving with Purpose: Exercise Strategies for Adults Over 30

It's quite simple really, if you've been reading this far you're well aware about the dynamic relationship between exercise, cortisol and insulin. This triumvirate holds the key to weight loss. Let's delve deeper and learn more about how the optimization of these hormones will help you reach your goals.

Either of these hormones are in a state known as equillibrium, as soon as one of them is disrupted they end up effecting your body, the moment cortisol the 'stress hormone' increases beyond an acceptable level, it hampers the rest of the bodies ability to regulate basic functions and processes. What does this mean? It means you can forget about healthy fat loss. These hormones all exist in a delicate balance that needs to be maintained either one cannot be greater or lower than the other.

Cortisol needs to be managed along with insulin to maintain healthy fat loss, the more elevated cortisol can insulin resistance which a state where the cells of the body become far less reponsive to the cues of insulin within it. This higher level of insulin resistance means that the body requires higher insulin levels to control blood sugar which means theres going to be more weight gain. When you manage cortisol, this balances out insulin levels to stay in one place keeping fat loss constant.

Working out or physical activity whether it involves a leisurely 45 minute walk, yoga or a heavy weight lifting session plays a crucial role in helping to manage cortisol levels. With the help of regular excersie your body becomes far more resilient to stress, which helps reduce cortisol spkes and as a result supports insulin sensitivty.

You need to consider activities such as brisk walks which are although gentle can be very effective in reducing cortisol, engaging in other low intensity steady state cardio activities such as jogging will also help release endorphins which are known as "feel-good" hormones, these counter act the effect of cortisol. Weight lifting is another powerful tool which builds muscle and serves as a shield against any hormonal imbalance.

It's important to keep in mind that overtraining can raise cortisol which can negate benefits of working out. This is why it's imperative to take rest days to maintain your homrone levels.

Exercise guides your hormones, you see the relationship between cortisol and insulin is not simply tied to your weight its also tied to your overall health. Lower cortisol levels will lead to getting higher quality sleep which will reduce inflammation as well as overal emotional and mental well being.

Let's look at the facts here, movement is a crucial aid to improve your horomonal health. Whatever it is, something as simple as stretching can be movement and can aid in your body's regulation of hormones. Every activity that you engage in adds to your body's ability to handle stress and manage cortisol in a productive and healthy fashion.

Hopefully this chapter empowers you with the knowledge that exercise is a powerful tool to help you in your journey of reaching your goals and improving your physical and emotional well-being.

Chapter 7

Beauty Sleep: Prioritizing Rest for Effective Weight Management

In this chapter, we will talk about the critical role that sleep plays in regulating mood, energy levels, and overall well-being. Adequate sleep, particularly around eight hours, is essential for lowering cortisol levels, the stress hormone. By reducing cortisol, the body gets a chance to reset and rebalance, enhancing both physical and mental health. Conversely, sleep deprivation elevates cortisol, adversely affecting insulin sensitivity and hindering fat loss efforts. Understanding and prioritizing sleep is crucial for achieving long-term health goals and maintaining a balanced lifestyle.

The benefits of deep sleep are a lot. One of the most significant advantages is the release of human growth hormone (HGH), which is vital for fat loss and muscle growth. HGH plays a crucial role in cell repair, muscle regeneration, and overall body composition. During deep sleep, the body enters a state of anabolic growth, where tissue repair and muscle growth are maximized. This process not only supports fat loss but also enhances physical performance and recovery, making it a cornerstone for athletes and fitness enthusiasts.

Deep sleep also bolsters the immune system. During this restorative phase, the body produces cytokines, proteins that combat inflammation and infection. These cytokines play a critical role in the immune response, helping the body to fend off pathogens and heal from injuries. Insufficient sleep impairs cytokine production, leaving the body more vulnerable to illnesses. Chronic sleep deprivation has been linked to an increased risk of various diseases, including cardiovascular disease, diabetes, and certain types of cancer. This underscores the importance of consistent, quality sleep for long-term health and disease prevention.

Establishing a consistent sleep routine is crucial for achieving restorative sleep. This involves creating a calming pre-sleep ritual, such as dimming the lights, turning off electronic screens, and reading a book. These activities signal to the body that it is time to wind down and prepare for rest. The blue light emitted by electronic screens can interfere with the production of melatonin, the hormone responsible for regulating sleep-wake cycles. By minimizing screen time before bed, you can enhance your body's natural ability to fall asleep and stay asleep.

Good sleep hygiene is equally important. This includes maintaining a comfortable sleep environment, sticking to a regular sleep schedule, and avoiding heavy meals or caffeine close to bedtime. A comfortable sleep environment typically involves a cool, dark, and quiet room, with a supportive mattress and pillows. Consistency in sleep schedules helps to regulate the body's internal clock, making it easier to fall asleep and wake up at the desired times. Avoiding stimulants like caffeine and heavy meals before bed can prevent disruptions in sleep patterns and promote more restful sleep.

Prioritizing sleep is important for both mental and physical health. Quality sleep nurtures and enhances the entire bodily system, including immune function and hormonal balance. Sleep is not a passive activity; it requires deliberate effort to meet the body's needs. Establishing a sleep routine and practicing good sleep hygiene are proactive steps that contribute to overall well-being. It also plays a crucial role in cognitive function. During sleep, the brain consolidates memories, processes information, and clears out toxins that accumulate during waking hours. This process is essential for maintaining cognitive sharpness, emotional stability, and overall mental health. Sleep deprivation, on the other hand, can lead to impaired memory, reduced concentration, and increased susceptibility to stress and anxiety.

We will further explore the importance of sleep in the coming chapters, as it is a fundamental component not only for fat loss but for overall well-being. Each night of good sleep is an investment in your health journey. By balancing cortisol levels, improving insulin sensitivity, and strengthening the immune system, sleep plays a crucial role in enhancing life quality and well-being.

Additionally, sleep has a huge impact on emotional regulation and mood stability. Adequate sleep helps to maintain a positive outlook and reduces the risk of mood disorders such as depression and anxiety. The restorative nature of sleep allows the brain to process emotions and reset, contributing to a more balanced and resilient mental state.

All things considered sleep is a vital aspect of health that influences numerous bodily functions. From hormonal balance and immune function to cognitive performance and emotional stability, sleep is a cornerstone of overall well-being. By understanding the importance of sleep and implementing strategies to improve sleep quality, you can enhance your health, support your fitness goals, and improve your quality of life. Sleep is not merely a passive state but an active investment in your future, and its benefits extend far beyond the realm of fat loss to encompass every aspect of physical and mental health.

Chapter 8

The Power Equation: Cultivating a Positive Weight Loss Mindset

Welcome to Chapter 8 of this unique and transformative book. In this chapter, we'll talk about a powerful formula that goes beyond just numbers: Routine + Discipline = Results. When you follow this formula, the results you achieve will boost your Confidence, helping you overcome challenges and achieve your goals.

Think of Routine as your map and Discipline as your compass. Routine helps you plan your actions, while Discipline keeps you on track. Establishing a Routine is like drafting a blueprint for success. This blueprint involves setting specific goals, planning your daily activities, and creating habits that align with your long-term objectives. Discipline, on the other hand, is the commitment to follow this blueprint, even when faced with obstacles or temptations. Together, Routine and Discipline become a natural part of your life.

Every small success builds your Confidence. Each pound lost and each workout completed strengthens your belief in your ability to succeed. This positive reinforcement makes it easier to maintain your Routine and Discipline. Results aren't just milestones; they're building blocks for a fortress of Confidence. With each achievement, your Confidence grows, enabling you to face challenges head-on and thrive in adversity.

Start by crafting your Routine. Picture yourself waking up early to exercise, taking cold showers to invigorate your body, and following a balanced schedule of meals, workouts, meditation, and leisure. These activities form your daily rhythm and contribute to your overall success.

Begin your day with a workout. This sets a positive tone for the rest of the day and boosts your energy levels. Cold showers are also another great idea. They might seem uncomfortable, but they offer benefits like improved circulation, boosted immunity, and better mood. They also symbolize your commitment to embracing challenges and growing stronger. Then, there's your meals. What you eat is fuel for your journey. Regular, balanced meals stabilize your blood sugar, keeping your energy levels steady and helping you stay focused. Meditation also helps reduce stress and improve mental clarity, supporting your overall well-being. Spend a few minutes each day in quiet reflection, focusing on your goals and progress.

Discipline is crucial for maintaining your Routine. It's the commitment to stick to your plan, even when it's difficult. This steadfastness ensures that your Routine becomes a natural part of your life. By willingly stepping into discomfort, such as taking cold showers or pushing through a tough workout, you build resilience and mental toughness. These qualities are essential for long-term success.

Creating a Routine involves more than just scheduling your activities. It requires thoughtful planning to ensure that each element of your day contributes to your overall goals. This means setting aside time for physical exercise, preparing nutritious meals, and incorporating activities that promote mental and emotional well-being. By doing so, you create a balanced and sustainable lifestyle that supports your weight loss journey.

Meditation and positive self-talk are crucial aspects of maintaining your Routine and Discipline. During quiet moments, reflect on your progress and speak to yourself kindly. Honesty and self-awareness will help you stay true to your goals and build Confidence. What you do when no one is watching is a reflection of your integrity and character. It's about being honest with yourself, acknowledging your strengths and weaknesses, and embracing transparency in your actions and intentions.

By following Routine + Discipline, you are taking intentional steps toward designing a fulfilling and healthy life. Implementing this equation requires a commitment to action. It means taking deliberate steps every day to follow your Routine and uphold your Discipline. This might involve setting specific goals, tracking your progress, and making adjustments as needed. The key is to remain consistent and dedicated, knowing that each small step brings you closer to your ultimate goal.

It is extremely important to remember that every choice you make brings you closer to your goals. Your Results will boost your Confidence, helping you face new challenges with strength and assurance. With Routine and Discipline as your guide, you can achieve remarkable transformations and live a life of purpose and vitality.

Step onto this path with intention. Every Routine you design and every act of Discipline you embrace brings you one step closer to your triumphant transformation. When you see your Results, Confidence will be your crown. It will be a sign of a life lived with purpose and power. Your journey towards healthy weight loss after 30 is highly dependent on your determination. By embracing the formula of Routine + Discipline = Results, you are laying the foundation for lasting success. Each Result achieved strengthens your Confidence, empowering you to tackle new challenges and continue growing. Let this chapter serve as a guide and inspiration as you walk your path, knowing that with Routine and Discipline, you can achieve remarkable transformations and live a life of fulfillment and vitality.

Chapter 9

Practical Tips for Real Life: Incorporating Weight Loss into Your Routine

When we talk about intermittent fasting and the ketogenic diet, there's one key thing that binds it all together. Discipline. It's your guiding force on this journey to a healthier you. Think of it as your North, keeping you on course even when the waters get rough. So, why is discipline so crucial? Here is why:

1. Consistency is Key

Discipline is the thread that weaves consistency into the fabric of your daily routine. When you commit to intermittent fasting and a ketogenic diet, it's the everyday dedication that yields the results you seek. Skipping a day here and there might seem inconsequential, but it can disrupt the momentum you've built. Imagine planting a garden and forgetting to water it every other day. Your plants would struggle to grow, right? The same applies to your health journey. Discipline ensures you show up every day, nurturing your body and mind with the right choices.

2. Overcoming Temptations

We live in a world filled with tempting treats and indulgent cravings. From the smell of freshly baked cookies wafting from a nearby bakery to the allure of a fast-food drive-thru, temptations are everywhere. Discipline acts as your shield against these seductive distractions. It's the inner voice that reminds you of your bigger goals, steering you away from sugary traps and empty calories. Picture it as a loyal friend who always has your best interests at heart, guiding you back on track when you veer off course.

3. Building Healthy Habits

The power of discipline lies in its ability to help you build healthy habits. Over time, the choices you make today become the habits that shape your future. Whether it's choosing a nourishing meal over a quick fix or sticking to your fasting schedule, discipline turns these choices into second nature. It's like training a muscle—the more you exercise it, the stronger it becomes. Eventually, these healthy habits will be ingrained in your daily routine, requiring less conscious effort and becoming an effortless part of your lifestyle.

4. Mental Resilience

Discipline isn't just about physical actions; it's about mental strength too. It's the ability to push through challenges, stay motivated, and bounce back from setbacks. This journey is as much about your mindset as it is about your body. When faced with obstacles, whether it's a busy schedule, social pressures, or emotional stress, discipline gives you the resilience to keep going. It's the mental fortitude that helps you stay focused on your goals, no matter what life throws your way.

5. Results and Confidence

Discipline leads to results, and results boost your confidence. The more you stick to your plan, the more progress you see. And that progress? It's a powerful confidence booster that spills over into all areas of your life. As you witness your transformation, you'll feel a renewed sense of self-assurance and empowerment. This newfound confidence will not only fuel your health journey but also positively impact your relationships, career, and overall well-being.

6. Long-Term Success

Discipline isn't a short-term fix; it's the cornerstone of long-term success. It's what separates those who achieve their goals from those who fall short. When you stick to your plan with unwavering discipline, you set the stage for lasting health and wellness. It's like building a house on a solid foundation—no matter how strong the storms, your house stands firm. With discipline, you're not just aiming for temporary results; you're creating a sustainable lifestyle that supports your health and happiness for years to come.

But let's be honest; discipline can be challenging at times. It requires commitment, focus, and determination. There will be days when you feel like giving up, when the comfort of old habits beckons, and when the results seem too slow. In these moments, remember the power of discipline. Visualize your goals, remind yourself of the progress you've made, and keep your eye on the prize.

So, when the going gets tough, embrace discipline as your ally. With it, there's no limit to what you can achieve on this journey to a healthier, happier you. Stick to the plan, and watch your transformation unfold. You've got this!

Chapter 10

Fasting: Rediscovering our Ancestral Rhythm

In this chapter, we will discuss the art of fasting in a bit more detail. Here, we will explore the evolution of fasting, from the 16:8 protocol to the mighty 36-hour fast. With meal plans that embrace the ketogenic diet, a moderate exercise routine, and a sleep regimen to lower cortisol, you'll set foot on a transformative journey.

The journey begins with the 16:8 protocol. Sixteen hours of fasting followed by an 8-hour eating window. During this period, your body learns to rely on stored fat for energy, promoting fat loss and improved insulin sensitivity. It's a lifestyle that seamlessly integrates with daily routines, providing a manageable and sustainable approach to intermittent fasting.

Initially, you might find the fasting hours challenging, but with time, your body adjusts. You'll notice increased mental clarity and energy levels as your body adapts to this new rhythm. It's a gentle introduction to the world of fasting, setting the stage for more extended fasting periods in the future.

As your body adapts, consider introducing 24-hour fasts 2-3 times a week. This more extended fast amplifies the benefits, allowing for deeper autophagy—a cellular cleansing process—and further insulin regulation. It's a conscious step forward, taking control of your metabolism and pushing your boundaries.

During these 24-hour fasts, you'll likely experience heightened mental clarity and a sense of accomplishment. Your body will further enhance its ability to utilize fat for fuel, making each fasting period easier and more effective. This phase is about exploring your limits and understanding how your body responds to extended fasting.

Once a week, do a 36-hour fast. This challenging yet transformative experience amplifies the metabolic benefits and fortifies your discipline. It's a powerful strategy to lower insulin, enhance fat loss, and reset your body's equilibrium.

The 36-hour fast is a true test of mental and physical strength. It requires preparation and mental fortitude, but the rewards are immense. You'll experience a deeper sense of cleansing, both physically and mentally. This practice teaches resilience, helping you understand the depth of your inner strength and determination.

A Ketogenic Feast: Meal Plans for Insulin Mastery

Pair your fasting journey with a ketogenic diet that keeps insulin levels in check. Here are a few meal plan examples:

1. **Classic Bacon and Eggs:** Scrambled or fried eggs with crispy bacon strips. Add sliced avocado for extra creaminess and healthy fats.
2. **Salmon and Asparagus:** Baked or grilled salmon fillet with roasted asparagus drizzled in olive oil and sprinkled with parmesan cheese.
3. **Caesar Salad with Grilled Chicken:** Romaine lettuce, grilled chicken, parmesan cheese, and Caesar dressing (use a keto-friendly dressing).

4 **Zucchini Noodles with Pesto and Cherry Tomatoes:** Spiralized zucchini noodles tossed in homemade pesto sauce with halved cherry tomatoes.

5 **Beef Stir-Fry with Broccoli:** Sliced beef cooked in a keto-friendly stir-fry sauce with broccoli, bell peppers, and mushrooms.

6 **Avocado and Bacon Stuffed Chicken:** Chicken breast stuffed with mashed avocado and wrapped in bacon, then baked until crispy.

7 **Cauliflower Fried Rice:** Cauliflower rice stir-fried with diced chicken or shrimp, mixed vegetables, and scrambled eggs in a keto-friendly stir-fry sauce.

8 **Caprese Salad with Mozzarella:** Sliced tomatoes, fresh mozzarella, and basil leaves drizzled with olive oil and balsamic vinegar reduction.

9 **Buttered Liver with Sautéed Spinach:** Beef liver, grass-fed butter, spinach, salt, and pepper.

10 **Creamy Spinach and Mushroom Beef:** Grilled beef served with a creamy spinach and mushroom sauce made with heavy cream and grated parmesan cheese.

11 **Avocado and Walnut Salad:** Mixed greens, sliced avocado, chopped walnuts, olive oil and balsamic vinegar for dressing, salt and pepper to taste.

12 **Buttered Brussels Sprouts with Almonds:** Fresh Brussels sprouts, 2 tablespoons of butter, sliced almonds, salt, and pepper to taste.

Remember to adjust portion sizes and ingredients to fit your specific macronutrient needs while following a ketogenic diet. These meal combinations provide a variety of flavors and textures to keep your keto journey enjoyable and satisfying.

The ketogenic diet prioritizes healthy fats, moderate proteins, and minimal carbohydrates. It's a fuel mix that complements fasting beautifully, ensuring you maintain energy levels and stay satiated during fasting periods.

Moderate Exercise Routine

Strength Training: Two to three times a week for muscle maintenance.

Cardio: Regular 30-minute sessions, such as brisk walks or cycling.

Yoga or Stretching: Enhances flexibility and promotes relaxation.

Picture that approaching deadline, the moment when you'll step on that scale and proudly meet your weight class—it's like a jolt of motivation that surges through you. It's a constant reminder that every single meal choice, every sweat-inducing workout, and every decision you make in the days leading up to the big event has a profound impact on your performance.

These principles are crucial whether you're chasing dreams in sports or aiming high in your personal and professional life. Discipline and routine are your secret weapons for achieving greatness.

This balanced approach keeps cortisol levels in check while promoting overall health. Always remember that sleep is a cornerstone. Prioritize 7 to 8 hours of quality sleep per night. A structured sleep regimen fosters hormonal harmony, ensuring cortisol stays at bay, and your fasting journey remains smooth.

Create a sleep sanctuary by maintaining a consistent sleep schedule, reducing screen time before bed, and creating a calming bedtime routine. Quality sleep is crucial for recovery, mental clarity, and overall well-being. It is extremely important to understand that fasting is a strategy deeply rooted in science. When you start fasting, your body will recalibrate, your metabolism will reset, and your confidence will soar. This will bring you closer to a life of vibrant health and empowered transformation.

Chapter 11

Eat the Cake

Welcome to a chapter that could hold the key to regaining control over your body after a sugar shock. You see, indulging in sugary or high-carbohydrate treats once in a while can sometimes lead to what we call a "sugar shock." But what exactly happens in your body when you consume all that sweetness?

At the cellular level, it's a bit like a storm brewing. Your blood sugar levels spike, setting off a cascade of events. Your pancreas kicks into high gear, releasing insulin to help your cells absorb all that sugar. This surge in insulin can lead to energy crashes and intense cravings for more sugar—ever felt those post-dessert cravings?

These sugar shocks can also throw your metabolism off balance. Your body starts storing excess sugar as fat, which can lead to weight gain. Furthermore, it can increase inflammation and oxidative stress, leaving your cells feeling a little battered.

Now, let's talk side effects. Bloating, fatigue, mood swings, and that notorious "sugar crash" are common after indulging in sugary delights. Your body's natural rhythm may be disrupted, affecting your sleep patterns and overall well-being.

But here's the uplifting part: your body is incredibly resilient. Just a few days of getting back on track with your fat-focused eating habits can work wonders. It's like hitting the reset button. Your insulin levels stabilize, cravings subside, and your body starts using stored fat for energy once again. Your metabolism regains its equilibrium, inflammation decreases, and your cells get a breather from oxidative stress. You'll find yourself feeling lighter, more energized, and back in control. It's amazing how quickly your body can bounce back when you give it the right fuel.

A little detour into sugar territory doesn't have to derail your progress. You have the power to reset, and it all begins with your next meal—a delicious, fat-focused meal that sets you back on the path to health and vitality.

I'm excited to share some fantastic news with you. Embracing this new way of eating, which revolves around understanding how to manipulate my insulin production, has given me a sense of freedom that's truly liberating. Yes, you read that right—freedom. While many people feel like slaves to their diets, I revel in the ability to enjoy all the incredible Brazilian dessert recipes passed down by my mother.

I've come to realize that my health and weight aren't about the traditional calorie-counting equation of "calories in versus calories out." It's about keeping my insulin levels in check. Armed with this knowledge, I can savor a slice of chocolate cake without a hint of guilt. Ice cream, cookies, pie, pizza—anything I desire is on the table.

Last Friday, I stepped onto the mats at the 2023 IBJJF Master Worlds in Las Vegas. Four intense matches led me to the final, where I fell short by the narrowest of margins and took home the silver. Naturally, I felt like celebrating being the 2023 vice world champion, and what better way than indulging in a scoop of ice cream and a generous slice of my mom's Chocolate Brigadeiro cake? Trust me, it tasted absolutely amazing.

That's not all. The very next day, I found myself munching on cookies and s'mores with my kids because, well, it was Labor Day. And here's the beauty of it all: there's no guilt, no remorse. Today, I'm right back on track, back to consuming healthy fats and keeping my insulin levels in check through fasting.

I won't sugarcoat it—pun intended. After those celebratory moments, I did feel a bit bloated and puffy, courtesy of a sugar rush. It's what happens when excess sugar finds its way into the cells. But here's the kicker: in just about three days, following my regimen, I can regain control over my insulin and return to my desired weight.

The good news is that life is full of moments worth celebrating—birthdays, weddings, family reunions, you name it. And when those occasions arise, you can go ahead and savor that cake, knowing that you now have the know-how to get right back on track. It's all about finding that balance and making informed choices.

Chapter 12

Unmasking Emotional Eating and Releasing Inner Blockages

In a world where emotional eating has become a global issue, it's time to dive into the heart of this complex matter. Why do people turn to food as a means to soothe their emotions, and what lies beneath the surface of this seemingly innocuous habit? The answers may surprise you.

Emotional eating, the act of using food as a coping mechanism for our feelings, often stems from a desire to find comfort, distraction, or even temporary relief from emotional turmoil. When life gets tough, when we face stress, sadness, or anxiety, the act of eating can become a refuge, offering a brief respite from our inner struggles. It's a way to numb the discomfort and fill the void left by unmet emotional needs.

It's not just about the food itself. Emotional eating is a complex dance between our emotional well-being and the choices we make. It's about the emotional blockages that we carry within us, often stemming from unresolved issues from our past, fears of the future, and a general sense of anxiety. These blockages can trap us in a cycle of emotional eating, where we consume food to mask our pain and frustration, only to feel guilt and regret afterward. Breaking free from this cycle demands that we take a closer look at our emotional landscape and acknowledge the presence of these blockages.

So, why is it so important to work on these emotional blockages? Because they are the keys to unlocking a healthier relationship with food and ourselves. By addressing these inner barriers, we gain a deeper understanding of why we eat our emotions away, and we equip ourselves with the tools needed to choose healthier coping mechanisms. It's a journey of self-discovery, healing, and personal growth, where we pave the way for emotional resilience, better decision-making, and an overall sense of well-being. Together, we'll explore the significance of unveiling our emotional blockages, confronting the fears of the future, and letting go of the burdens of the past. It's a transformative path toward a life where food is no longer a crutch for our emotions but a nourishing source of fuel and pleasure.

In our exploration of emotional eating, it's vital to underscore the significance of unraveling the unsolved issues that often trace their roots back to our childhood. Each of us carries within ourselves a tapestry of experiences and emotions woven together from encounters with parents, teachers, religious leaders, friends, and countless others. These encounters have left their mark, and they've created a tapestry of hundreds of blockages. These blockages are the moments in our lives that elicited powerful emotions, and our intelligent brains have learned to shield us from these feelings, even if they no longer serve us.

These unresolved issues, these emotional blockages, hold tremendous power over our choices, including the way we turn to food to cope with emotions. They are the whispers from our past that influence our present decisions, often without our conscious awareness. To break free from emotional eating, it's imperative that we first identify these blockages, these emotional knots that have been silently shaping our relationship with food. When we confront these deep-rooted issues, we begin the process of untangling their grip on our lives.

It's a process of personal transformation, one that opens the door to a life of prosperity and abundance. By releasing these inner blockages, we free ourselves from the shackles of emotional eating, unlocking our potential to flourish. As we heal and grow, our newfound emotional freedom cascades into every aspect of our existence, touching not only our lives but also the lives of those around us. We become a source of positivity, inspiration, and resilience, overflowing with an abundance of well-being that knows no bounds. The path to emotional freedom is a profound one, and it is yours to embark upon, illuminating a future where food is no longer a crutch, but a source of nourishment and delight.

Chapter 13

Success Stories: Inspiring Journeys of Weight Loss After 30

Before we conclude our journey, let's take a look at some inspirational stories from different people.

Lola Pinto

"After a series of turbulence in our lives, everything in our body undergoes a transformation. An excessive dose of adrenaline followed by stress often results in thyroid dysfunction. There you have it!

Your body quickly starts to store fat, causing a sudden increase in weight. It was then that I found myself in a situation where I needed to return to my physical activities. I felt that my body was crying out for me to return to the active lifestyle I had since childhood. I began practicing jiu-jitsu at the age of 56. In parallel, I adopted a ketogenic diet, of which I was already a fan back when I used to dance in my adolescence. Of course, over the years, I have gathered more information about its health benefits.

In three months, I transformed into a different person with a new body. The whole process of eating every 24 to 48 hours provided me with better physical conditioning, allowing me to train twice a day for six days a week. That's when I embarked on my journey in jiu-jitsu, a discipline that made me realize how capable I am of overcoming challenging situations without injuring myself. This opened my eyes to the importance of my health, which is, in reality, our most valuable asset. Our body is what carries our soul through life to fulfill a mission. I felt an obligation to keep my body and mind in sync to face this challenge—losing 30 pounds and competing in my first championship.

I demonstrated a lot of determination and discipline throughout the process of consuming a diet based on healthy fats and protein. It represents a true transformation and a new approach to life. The initial sensation is an increase in self-esteem that guides you toward success, followed by an improvement in your health. Everything aligns perfectly. I found myself in a state of pure balance—Mente Sana, Corpo Sano (a healthy mind in a healthy body). This diet instilled in me a sense of self-assessment and a heightened awareness of every food I consume as a form of natural medicine. I no longer feel a compulsive need to eat, but rather a desire to nourish the cells that keep me alive."

Renata Pinto

"After gaining 65 pounds during my twin pregnancy, I faced the challenge of shedding excess weight and dealing with saggy skin. Despite following the recommended guidelines, the post-pregnancy journey was tough. It took six months post-breastfeeding for me to focus on reclaiming my pre-baby self. Skeptical about strict diets, I turned to my husband's advice, and the transformation was remarkable. With enjoyable, real food and occasional cheat meals, I effortlessly shed 25 pounds in just four months. Not only did I reach my goal weight, but the saggy skin disappeared too. Now, I feel healthier, confident, and ready to enjoy every moment with my three kids. Weight loss isn't just about appearance; it's about being healthy for my family's future."

Efraim Silva

"My journey began at Ninja's house, watching his three children eating bacon. I became concerned that he would harm the kids, so I asked, and Ninja gave me a lesson and motivated me to read some books like "The Obesity Code." Then, I realized that my life was about to be transformed, and in reality, I was living with numerous health issues, thinking I was healthy. I had to take stomach medications because otherwise, I would be in pain all day. At night, I had to sleep with the CPAP machine; I had sleep apnea, a severe allergy that triggered asthma. I had to take antihistamines, and I had a lot of chronic pain that I thought was due to age and capoeira. So, in three months of adopting this lifestyle, removing sugar, carbohydrates, and vegetable oils from my life, my life turned from water to wine, and all health problems disappeared. Then, I started helping everyone in my life. Without Ninja's motivation and teachings, nothing would have happened, so I am very grateful. I could talk for a long time, but I'll keep it brief, as we can do a live podcast about this."

Nair Moraes

"It is with great pleasure and satisfaction that I report an event that changed my life forever. It was a great learning experience, which I recommend to everyone.

I learned how to replace foods to achieve a healthier lifestyle. It took me 58 years, but I did it. I lost 8.5 kilos in 45 days, and I realized that only I could change my life and that no one could do it for me. It's really worth it; you'll see how much your body and health have improved."

Olavo Gonçalves

"This is real... pork rinds, ribs, pancetta, bacon, fried egg... Everything is part of my life. I went from 74 kilos to 65 kilos, which was my barracks weight, without high cholesterol, without any problems. I am 63 years old and completely healthy."

Jorge Latuf

"I discovered that I had diabetes in 2014. At first, it was pre-diabetes, but as time went by, and given the difficulties in being able to correctly follow medical instructions regarding medication and nutrition, combined with physical exercise. The disease lasted until it reached grade 2, which persisted until mid-2022 when I started having to use insulin.

However, after guidance from my nephew, Felipe Ninja, who is dedicated to studying the subject, I started using a fat-based diet, with complete abstinence from carbohydrates, combined with physical exercise. I had a significant regression in my glucose levels, which improved my health, even at 70 years of age. In mid-September 2023, it allowed me to completely eliminate insulin from my daily medication, as well as eliminate a third of the complementary medication I use.

I lead a normal life, practicing physical exercise and having low sugar levels in my body."

Rui Kapoeira

"I want to express my deepest gratitude to my friend, Ninja, whose wisdom and support were fundamental in my weight loss journey. His valuable information and constant encouragement helped me achieve my goals and transform my life. I am eternally grateful for his friendship!"

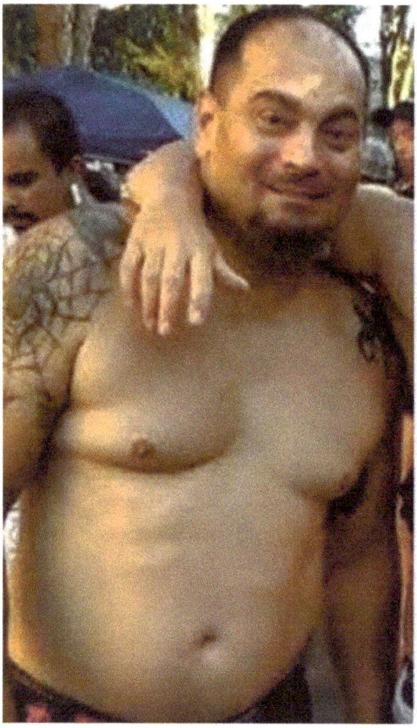
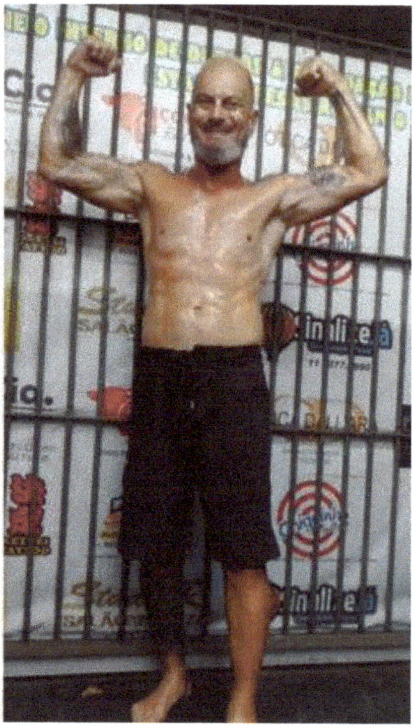

Author's Note

Dear Reader,

Firstly, a heartfelt thank you for taking the time to journey through the pages of my book on weight loss after 30. Your commitment to understanding and embracing a healthier lifestyle is truly commendable.

Completing this book is an accomplishment. It marks the beginning of a transformative path toward a healthier, more vibrant lifestyle. I want to commend you for investing in yourself and your well-being. You've taken the first step toward a future filled with vitality, longevity, and a sense of well-deserved achievement.

Remember, change doesn't happen overnight, and the journey to a healthier life requires dedication and discipline. Trust the process, and don't be discouraged by setbacks. Each small step you take contributes to a more robust, healthier future. Your body will thank you, and you'll reap the benefits not only physically but also mentally and emotionally.

Embrace the remarkable changes that lie ahead. Picture a life filled with energy, resilience, and a sense of well-being. It's not just about shedding pounds; it's about gaining a life full of joy, vitality, and countless memorable moments.

As you continue your journey, hold onto the belief that healthy longevity is within reach. The benefits you'll experience are unparalleled – improved energy levels, mental clarity, and a profound sense of accomplishment. Trust the process, stay disciplined, and let the remarkable transformation unfold.

Thank you again for joining me on this empowering experience. May your path be filled with health, happiness, and a life truly well-lived.

With gratitude,
Luis Felipe Ninja Pinto

www.ingramcontent.com/pod-product-compliance
Lightning Source LLC
LaVergne TN
LVHW051932051126
851857LV00020B/2082
* 9 7 8 1 9 6 4 9 1 3 7 0 4 *